Aromatherapy

A Guide to the Healing Powers of Aromatherapy and Essential Oils

Table of Contents

Introduction

Imagine a world where you cannot smell anything; life would be so weird, boring, and stressful. Of course, there are smells we would rather not smell like carcasses, rotting food, and bodily waste, but there are also many other wonderful smells like spices, flowers, trees, and freshly cooked food. These smells can remind us of good times and invoke in us a sense of wellbeing.

Though under-utilized by most of us, your sense of smell is one of the best methods of boosting moods, encouraging good health, and relieving stress. Aromatherapy is one such method through which we can make use of this sense. Aromatherapy makes use of naturally extracted elements like essential and natural oils which not only refresh the mind but can also cure and heal various health problems.

What exactly does Aromatherapy refer to?

Aromatherapy is the art and science of using volatile oils derived from plants for psychological and physical well-being. Essential oils are the most commonly used oils in aromatherapy. This is because of their innumerable benefits, which you will learn more about later. In aromatherapy, different essential oils are used to achieve different therapeutic results.

How does it work?

Aromatherapy works when you inhale certain scents that trigger hypothalamus stimulation. The hypothalamus is the part of the brain responsible for regulating important bodily functions like sleep and emotional responses. When the scent stimulus reaches the hypothalamus, it travels through the limbic system into the part of the brain that is crucial for memory — the hippocampus. This helps the body and mind react to the healing scents of aromatherapy, thus imparting a sense of well-being.

The Origins of Aromatherapy

There is some debate over when and where aromatherapy was discovered first. If you didn't know, aromatherapy has been in use for thousands of years, even though it only came to be known as aromatherapy somewhere in the 19th century. Many people have used aromatherapy for their well-being without consciously knowing it was aromatherapy.

Aromatherapy is believed by most to be of Chinese origin. It was around 2000 BC when Chinese civilizations discovered the medicinal properties of black pepper. Egyptians are believed to have been using aromatherapy at around the same time as the Chinese. Egyptians used an infusion method to extract the oils from aromatic plants such as cinnamon, nutmeg, cedarwood, clove, and myrrh. They were experts in preserving the flesh by using aromatics for embalming. They also applied fragrant oils after bathing.

From Egyptians, aromatherapy is said to have been passed on to the Greeks. The Greeks continued using aromatic oils in water for fragrances and as a specific distillation and incense to enhance the prophetic abilities of the Oracles. They also use them for medicinal purposes. After Greece, it moved to Rome. The Romans made use of their medical knowledge from the Greeks and increased the different applications of essential oils. They used the essential oils to massage and oil themselves after bathing. Persians and Indians also used aromatherapy thousands of years ago.

Backed by a rich history, it wasn't until the 19th century that scientists from Europe and Britain began research on aromatherapy products to understand their effects on mind and body. Rene Gattefosse, a French chemist, quickly immersed his hand in lavender oil after burning it in his laboratory. He was shocked with how quickly the burn healed. He thereafter began his research into the healing powers of essential oils. He even published a book on the antimicrobial effects of essential oils in 1937. He is the one who coined the term "Aromatherapy" before it became conventional terminology. Other French scientists discovered Gattefosse's research and improved on it. They began experimenting with essential oils and developed unique methods of applying them to the skin. These scientists worked together and combined techniques to create the version of Aromatherapy that is in use now all over the world.

Essential Benefits of Aromatherapy

Several studies have proven that aromatherapy can serve as an aid for various ailments, besides just relaxing your body. Aromatherapy has endless benefits available to everyone. Here are some of the impressive benefits that aromatherapy can provide:

Improve Sleep Quality

Do you have trouble with sleeping? If your answer is "yes", then Aromatherapy is a solution that you should try. Essential oils, when topically used in aromatherapy, help stimulate the limbic system in the brain. In effect, this calms and relaxes your mind and body, leading you into a deep sleep. And when you wake up, you feel refreshed.

Help Relieve Chronic Asthma

If you suffer from consistent coughing and chronic wheezing because of chronic asthma, aromatherapy can provide good relief. When used wisely and under professional care, it can free your lungs from discomfort and irritation.

Improve Skin Complexion

Aromatherapy has proven to be a great treatment for many skin conditions. Some skin types like dry and flaky can cause premature wrinkling if left untreated. For this reason, using essential oils can help maintain moist, youthful, and balanced skin. Aromatherapy also improves more serious skin conditions, like eczema and psoriasis.

Improve Mood and Relieves Stress

Rosemary and basil oils are the most commonly used essential oils to boost mood and offer feelings of contentment, thus easing depression. These oils have proven to regulate the production of the stress hormone, cortisol. Therefore, the regular use of these oils can help relieve stress, induce relaxation, and prevent anxiety.

Treats Bladder Infections

Aromatherapy can quickly treat bladder infections when correctly administered. The most commonly used essential oils for treating bladder infections include tea tree, chamomile, sandalwood, and juniper berry. To avoid harmful side effects, use trained aromatherapy techniques to administer them correctly. Common methods for getting rid of a bladder infection include applying the essential oil in a compress over the bladder or taking an aromatherapy bath.

Treat Nausea and Digestion Problems

Do you suffer from digestion problems like stomach pain, intestinal gas, gastroenteritis, belching, and nausea? If you didn't know, aromatherapy can help to relieve all of the above! Aromatherapy signals the brain in the initial stage of digestion that food is on the way. As a result, the brain stimulates the release of important digestive juices that help ease stomach problems.

Lessen the symptoms of PMS

Premenstrual syndrome is a condition that most women struggle with during their premenopausal lifetime. These women go through physical and emotional problems brought about by symptoms of PMS. Aromatherapy has proven to be a powerful reliever of these symptoms. Therefore, if you experience severe symptoms around your period, aromatherapy might be the perfect solution for you. Treatment can involve taking an aromatic bath or getting a massage with essential oils.

Pain Management

Clove bud oil is commonly used by people to reduce body pain. It has proven to be a very potent essential oil in pain management. Just ensure that you use it with care and dilute it properly first if you want to use it as a lotion for massage.

Heal Wounds

Tea tree and helichrysum oils have proven to be effective in the management of wounds if correctly used. Clean the wound first with tea tree oil, and then apply helichrysum essential oil on the areas near the wound. To promote faster and safer healing, avoid applying the oil directly to the wound.

As you can see, aromatherapy is a legitimate and effective alternative healing therapy for many different conditions. Why take countless pills that may contain harmful chemicals if you can enjoy a gentle but natural substitute that will ease many illnesses and concerns from your body? Nowadays, many healthcare professionals are prescribing aromatherapy for a variety of ailments, including both physical and emotional problems. The benefits listed in this introduction are just the beginning. We are going to look more into the healing powers of aromatherapy and essential oils in the following chapters. Let's dive in!

Chapter One: Guidelines for Using Essential Oils

Anyone can buy essential oils and start using them right away. However, if you want to go deeper and explore aromatherapy safely, learning how to use them systematically is a wise move. It takes just a short amount of time to integrate essential oils into your daily routine; it only requires a bit of basic knowledge, patience, and a willingness to try something new.

Before you start aromatherapy, you must know what you need and want to achieve with essential oils first. Also, you need to understand how to use these oils in a way that is both safe and effective. In simple terms, you need to follow some guidelines and create a plan that works for you. The approach discussed below will help you do just that:

Determine Your Needs

To decide on which essential oils to use, you must first determine your needs. There are two significant questions you should ask yourself:

1. Why have you chosen to try aromatherapy?

2. What do you want to achieve by using essential oils?

Once you have the answers to these questions, then you're ready to go. Some of your reasons for using essential oils may be:

- To naturally treat particular ailments
- To increase energy naturally and improve your emotions

- To enjoy quality sleep without reaching for sleeping pills
  - To reduce household chemical use
  - Because you are interested in a holistic approach to health

Shopping for Essential Oils

Understand that many brands sell essential oils, but not all brands are equal. Therefore, when you shop for essential oils, do your best to find high-quality ones. Don't just be convinced by buzzwords; check and ensure that what they are selling you is pure natural essential oil. To select the best quality essential oils, use the following tips:

- Research the companies that produce them and read consumers' reviews.
- Look for key labelling components and botanical names.
- Note the country of origin for the essential oil you are buying.
- Avoid purchasing essential oils from street vendors, craft shows, or other limited-time events.
- Look for a brand that has existed for a long time and offers a wide range of products.
- Avoid essential oils packaged in clear glass and plastic containers. To avoid oxidizing effects of light, essential oils should be packaged in dark-colored glass or lined aluminum containers.
- Cheap is expensive; avoid essential oils that seem too cheap.
- Always research before purchasing essential oils and be on the lookout for anything that sounds too good to be true. Above all, listen and trust your intuition.

Use your Essential Oils Safely

Essential oils are natural but extremely powerful. Since they are highly potent and concentrated, it is important to approach working with them respectfully and safely. Therefore, for you to benefit from these versatile oils, you need to be aware of safety issues, recommended dilutions, and methods of application.

Safety precautions/ Guidelines for safe and effective use

- Always use only pure essential oils that are derived from plants, not the ones manufactured in laboratories.
- Avoid applying undiluted essential oils directly to your skin.
- Always dilute essential oils in a carrier oil.
- Always check for sensitivities to essential oils or carrier products by patch testing before applying them to the entire region.
- Take caution with photosensitivity and use essential oils that result in it with care. They may cause irritation and uneven pigmentation to the skin.
- Avoid or use with caution those essential oils that irritate the mucous membranes.
- Alternate the essential oils you use.
- Store all essential oils out of the reach of children.
- Be very cautious when using essential oils to treat your pets. You may like to use a ratio designed for children, as pets like dogs and cats have much thinner skin than people.
- Overexposure to essential oils may cause nausea, headache, skin irritation, or emotional unease. Try as much as possible to avoid it.
- Do not take essential oils orally. They are likely to cause burning to the mucous membrane of your mouth.

- In case of any reaction, see your doctor immediately.
- Avoid applying essential oils near your eyes.
- Do not apply essential oils to broken skin or open wounds.
- Be cautious about using essential oils while pregnant.

Methods of Application

There are different ways to apply essential oils. Your choice depends entirely on what you are using them for. Most of these applications require the use of only a minimal amount of oil.

Massage- Essential oils can be applied directly to the skin through a massage. This is one of the most beneficial methods of applying aromatherapy, as it combines the powerful effects of essential oils with the therapeutic touch of massage. To aid application, essential oils must be diluted in a carrier oil like sweet almond, grapeseed, or olive oil in a specific dilution ratio.

Bathing- This is one of the easiest ways of using essential oils at home. You just need to add a few drops of essential oils to the bathtub. The heat and steam empower and disperse the oils which are later absorbed in the skin and through inhalation.

Foot Bath- A warm foot bath of essential oils after a hard day is so relaxing. A foot bath is great for blisters and tired feet. Simply dilute your essential oils in the recommended ratio and put a few drops into a large bowl of warm water. Soak your feet and relax for 10-15 minutes.

Compresses- Compresses are applied when you need to put the oil directly on the affected area. Simply add diluted essential oil to a bowl of water, soak a cotton cloth in, wring out excess water and wrap the affected area.

Diffusion- This is one of the most interesting ways to get the best value of essential oils and make your home smell lovely at the same time. Diffusers do just that, they diffuse essential oils into the air of a room leaving it with a lovely scent.

Inhalation- This is the quickest way to get essential oils into the body and get an immediate effect. The different ways to use the inhalation method include diffusion using a nebulizer to spray a fine mist into the air, opening the bottle and smelling it, inhaling the steam of vapors from oils put into hot water, applying a few drops of the oils on a tissue and smelling it directly, or rubbing few drops between your palms, and cupping over your nose.

How to Mix Essential Oils

To get the therapeutic benefits of essential oils, you must dilute them correctly. The most effective way of diluting these oils is using carrier oils like almond, apricot, sesame, grapeseed, and olive oil.

In most aromatherapy applications, a dilution of 2 percent is considered the safest and most effective. This translates to 2 drops of essential oil per 100 drops of carrier oil. This applies to various types of aromatherapies, however, in some individuals and situations, you may require a lower or slightly higher percentage, though the dilution percentage rarely goes to 3 percent no matter the purpose.

For pregnant women, the elderly, people with health concerns, and children, a dilution percentage of between 1 and 1.5 are the most recommended. For massage oils, use 1 percent or about 6 drops of essential oil to an ounce of carrier oil. This is because a lot of oil is needed during the massage. In aromatherapy, more is not better. And in fact, using too much essential oil will cause adverse or opposite results.

You can also create a safe and effective aromatherapy mixture through blending. There are two reasons for creating your aromatherapy blends: to enjoy a pleasurable personalized scent and to get the therapeutic benefits that come with the use of essential oils. When combining essential oils in a therapeutic blend, keep it simple if you are a beginner. Use recipes when creating your blend.

Storing your Essential Oils

Proper storage of essential oils preserves their therapeutic properties, and also increases their shelf life. Even though essential oils don't go rancid the same way carrier oils do, they lose their freshness and potency when exposed to heat and light. Of all the essential oils, citrus, fir, and pine oils have the shortest shelf life, so make use of them when they are at their freshest. The good news is that you may extend their shelf life by refrigerating and keeping them out of sunlight. Keeping your essential oils in a cool, dark area with a stable temperature is the best way to store them. Never store your essential oils in direct sunlight, as they will get oxidized and cause rapid deterioration.

Key takeaways
- Before starting aromatherapy, have a simple goal and purpose in mind.
- Always do your research before shopping for your essential oils.
- Avoid purchasing essential oils from street vendors, craft shows, or other limited-time events.

- Always dilute your essential oils in a carrier oil using a correct ratio.
- Do not take essential oils orally.
- Never store your essential oils in direct sunlight.

Chapter Two: Commonly Used Essential Oils & Carrier Oils

Aromatherapy is widely used in both beauty industries and medical practices. For this reason, there are many essential oils on the market that are proven to work well for both the body and mind. This chapter explores the most commonly used essential oils, stating their categories, Latin names, origin, and what they blend with best. It does not include all the essential oils, but the list is quite comprehensive. Before we dive too deeply into this, let's look at the different categories of essential oils that exist!

Categories of Essential Oils

The aroma of the essential oils is important in making your experience pleasant. With that said, we have three categories of essential oils. They include top notes, middle notes, and base notes. This classification is based on how long the natural scent lasts. Every essential oil fits into at least one of these categories. Essential oil note level classification is further explained below:

Top Notes

This is the strongest group of essential oils. The oils in this category are all sharp-smelling, stimulating, penetrating, uplifting and volatile. Their aroma can last up to 24 hours. When you place them on your skin, you experience either a cold or hot sensation. Always use fewer drops of top notes in your formula.

Middle Notes

Middle note essential oils act as equalizers in formulas, thus controlling the intensity of the more active essential oils. They have scents that most people like, and therefore they often make up the bulk of the formula. Their aromas can last up to three days.

Base Notes

Essential oils that fall into this category have aromas that last the longest. The depth and intensity of these oils deepen and enrich the blend in formulas. Most base notes can penetrate the skin more thoroughly than other oil types. Their aroma may not be noticed upon initial contact with the nose, but it results in an aromatic smell when left on the skin.

List of Commonly Used Essential Oils

1. **Cedarwood (*Cedrus atlantica*)** Cedarwood essential oil falls under the base note category of essential oils. It belongs to a family known as Pinaceae which is found in North America. Native Americans traditionally used it to preserve their dead. It is extracted through steam distillation. It blends well with essential oils like bergamot, cypress, jasmine, juniper, neroli, and rosemary.

2. **Carrot (*Daucus carota*)** This falls under the middle note category of essential oils. This wild carrot is a vegetable belonging to the Umbelliferae family, and is grown primarily for aromatherapy in England. The essential oil is extracted from its roots and seeds. It blends

well with essential oils like chamomile German, cypress, lavender, and lemon.

3. **Basil (*Ocinum bacilicum*)** Basil essential oil is in the top note category and belongs to the Labiate family whose origin is Asia. Basil is among the herbs that are regularly used in cooking. Basil is a powerful herb with amazing therapeutic properties. This essential oil is extracted from the whole plant. It blends well with essential oils like bergamot, fennel, geranium, grapefruit, juniper, and lavender.

4. **Camphor (*Cinnamonum camphora*)** Camphor essential oil falls under the middle note category. It is extracted from the Asian evergreen tree that belongs to the Lauraceae family. It blends well with essential oils like clary sage, cypress, eucalyptus, frankincense, and sandalwood.

5. **Bergamot (*Citrus bergamia*)** Bergamot essential oil falls in the category of top-note essential oils. The Bergamot tree belongs to the liutaceae family and was first grown in Italy. The oil is extracted from its ripe fruit peel. Other essential oils that blend well with it are cypress, jasmine, lavender, neroli, patchouli, and ylang-ylang.

6. **Benzoin (*Styrax benzoin*)** Benzoin essential oil falls in the base note category. The tree belongs to the Styraceae family whose origin is Thailand and Sumatra. Other essential oils that blend well with it include carrot, cedarwood, neroli, petitgrain, rose, and sandalwood.

7. **Cinnamon (*Cinnamonum zeylanicum*)** Cinnamon essential oil is in the category of top note oils. The cinnamon tree belongs to the Lauraceae family. It was first grown in Madagascar, India, and Sri Lanka. It blends well with essential oils like chamomile German, clove, fennel, and geranium.

8. **Cypress (*Cupressis sempervirens*)** Cypress essential oil falls in the middle note category. The tree belongs to the Cupressaceae family. It is grown naturally in German and France. This essential oil is extracted from the flowers, leaves, and twigs. Other essential oils that blend well with it are chamomile German, juniper, lavender, parsley, pine, and sandalwood.

9. **Fennel (*Foeniculum vulgare*)** Fennel essential oil falls in the middle note category. The herb belongs to the Umbelliferae family, and it is grown worldwide. It blends well with essential oils like basil, cinnamon, geranium, lavender, rose, and sandalwood.

10. **Hyssop (*Hyssopus officinalis*)** Hyssop belongs to the Labiate family. The essential oil falls under the middle note category. It is a very strong herb and produces an exceptionally potent oil. The essential oil is extracted from its leaves and flower tops. Other essential oils that blend well with it include benzoin, chamomile Roman, clary sage, lavender, palma-rosa, rosemary, and sage.

11. **Jasmine (*Jasminum officinale*)** Jasmine essential oil is of the base note category. The bush belongs to the Oleaceae family, and it is cultivated in West Africa, China, and France. The essential oil is extracted from its flowers. It blends well with most essential oils.

12. **Juniper (*Juniperus communis*)** Juniper essential oil belongs to the middle category. The bush is of Cupressaceae family and originated in Europe. The essential oil is extracted from its dried berries. Other essential oils that blend well with it include benzoin, clary sage, clove, cypress, lavender, and sandalwood.

13. **Lime (*Citrus aurantifolia*)** This is a top-note essential oil. The lime tree belongs to the Rutaceae family. The essential oil is extracted from the rind of lime fruit. It was first cultivated in California and Florida. It blends well with essential oils like bergamot, jasmine, mandarin, and orange.

14. **Marjoram (*Origanum marjorana*)** Marjoram essential oil falls in the middle note essential oil category. It is extracted from leaves and flower tops. It was first grown in Egypt. It blends well with essential oils like benzoin, bergamot, cypress, lavender, petitgrain, and rosemary.

15. **Melissa (*Melissa officinalis*)** Melissa essential oil falls in the middle note category of essential oils. It is commonly referred to as balm oil. Melissa herb belongs to the Labiate family. The oil is extracted from its leaves. Other essential oils that blend well with it include geranium, lavender, neroli, and ylang-ylang.

16. **Neroli (*Citrus bagaradia*)** This is a top-note essential oil. It belongs to a family of trees known as Rutaceae. The essential oil is extracted from the flower petals of the tree. It originated in Italy. It blends well with essential oils like benzoin, bergamot, clary sage, geranium, jasmine, lavender, and orange.

17. **Niaouli (*Melaleuca viridiflora*)** Niaouli is among the top-note essential oils. This bush belongs to the family known as Myrtaceae. The essential oil is extracted from its leaves and twigs. It works well with essential oils like clary sage, eucalyptus, geranium, lavender, myrrh, patchouli, and tea tree.

18. **Myrrh (*Commiphora myrrha*)** Myrrh is a base note essential oil. The tree belongs to a family known as Burseraceae. Myrrh essential oil is extracted from the bark of the tree as a gum resin. It blends well with essential oils like basil, camphor, cypress, eucalyptus, lavender, niaouli, and thyme.

19. **Parsley (*Petroselinum sativum*)** Parsley falls under the base note category of essential oils. Parsley herb belongs to the Labiate family. The essential oil is extracted from the seeds of the herb. It can blend well with essential oils like cypress, geranium, grapefruit, and sage.

20. **Palmarosa (*Cymbopogon martini*)** Palmarosa is a middle note essential oil. The grass belongs to the Graminae family. Its oil is extracted from the whole plant. It blends perfectly with essential oils like carrot, chamomile Roman, hyssop, patchouli, and sandalwood.

21. **Spearmint (*Mentha spicata*)** This oil is among the top-note essential oils. The herb is from the Labiate family. The essential oil is extracted from the flower tops and leaves of the plant. Other essential oils that blend perfectly with it are basil, lavender, parsley, and petitgrain.

22. **Orange (*Citrus aurantium*)** The orange tree belongs to the family we call Rutaceae. It was first grown in China. The essential oil is among the top note category, and it is extracted from the rind of the fruit. It blends well with essential oils like cedarwood, geranium, ginger, lemon, lime, neroli, and petitgrain.

23. **Violet leaves (*Viola odorata*)** Violet leaves essential oil is in the middle note category. The plant belongs to the Labiate family. The oil is extracted from its leaves. The best quality of this oil comes from England. It blends perfectly with essential oils like benzoin, carrot, cypress, fennel, neroli, and rose bulgar/maroc.

24. **Ylang-ylang (*Cananga odorata*)** Essential oil from this tree has the characteristics of all three categories. However, the base note category outweighs the rest. Ylang-ylang tree belongs to the family known as Annonaceae. Its oil is extracted from its blooming flowers. Other essential oils that blend well with it include bergamot, clary sage, frankincense, jasmine, lavender, lemon, and neroli.

25. **Sage (*Salvia officinalis*)** Sage essential oil falls in the top note category. The herb belongs to the Labiate family. The essential oil is extracted from the flower tops and sun-dried leaves of the herb. It blends well with lemongrass, sandalwood, and violet leaf oil.

26. **Sandalwood (*Santalum album*)** Sandalwood essential oil is a base note oil. The tree belongs to a family known as the Santalaceae. The oil is extracted from its heart's center, which is the reason for its limited availability and high cost. It can blend perfectly with

benzoin, cypress, frankincense, juniper, neroli, palmarosa, rose bulgar, rose maroc, and ylang-ylang.

The other commonly used essential oils that top the list include lavender, thyme, peppermint, lemon, clove, German chamomile, tea tree, rosemary, patchouli, lemongrass, geranium, frankincense, eucalyptus, and clary sage. You must wonder why we have said nothing about them, yet they top the list. Don't worry, we are going to look more into their profiles in the next chapter!

Carrier/ Base Oils

A carrier oil is a substance that is used to dilute and "carry" the essential oil into the body. The terms "carrier oil' and "base oil" are used interchangeably, so do not confuse "base oil" with "base note". All essential oils are mixed with a carrier oil before use. Each carrier oil has its own unique reaction to the skin, hair, and nails, and this is one reason why aromatherapy can be complicated. Some carrier oils like avocado and hazelnut penetrate faster while others like wheat germ nourish the skin. This should not overwhelm you; fortunately, most of the carrier oils react in a manner that is quite similar.

List of Carrier Oils

List of Carrier Oils	
Almond oil	Apricot kernel oil
Castor oil	Cocoa butter
Avocado oil	Borage seed oil
Arnica oil	Baobab oil
Hazelnut oil	Wheat germ oil
Rosehip oil	Black seed oil
Corn oil	Evening primrose oil
Grapeseed oil	Jojoba oil
Olive oil	Peanut oil
Safflower oil	Sesame oil
Coconut oil	Argan oil

Soya bean oil	Sunflower oil
Black cumin seed oil	Calendula oil
Carrot seed oil	Camellia oil
Cucumber seed oil	Cupuacu butter

As you familiarize yourself with aromatherapy treatments, you find that some carrier oils are easier to work with than others. Have it in mind that not everyone will have the same reaction to the different carrier oils. Therefore, performing a patch test is the best way to find what suits you. This is done by simply applying a small amount of oil to a small area of skin and waiting to see if there is a reaction.

Chapter Three: The Profile of Conventional Essential Oils

Nowadays, finding aromatherapy products is very easy. While high accessibility is on the list of positives for veterans, novice users and some curious consumers end up using essential oils incorrectly, which can expose them and their loved ones to potential skin irritations and allergic reactions. Knowledge is very key to safe essential oil use.

This chapter gives you the profiles of the 14 conventional essential oils that should top your list of the 'must-haves', providing you with the Latin name of each essential oil, its description, their healing properties, method of application, and important safety information on their use.

1. **Lavender Essential Oil (*Lavandula angustifolia*)**
   This incredibly popular essential oil is renowned for its ability to calm the mind while aiding deep relaxation and supporting restful sleep. It has all kinds of benefits. It can also be used in some first-aid treatments, thanks to its healing and regenerative properties. For skincare, it is a great option as it works for all skin types. It can help relieve minor skin irritations and support healthy skin. Inhaling it has been found to help with alleviating headaches.

Precautions:

- Excessive use of lavender oil can cause allergic reactions.

Application Methods:

- Inhalation- inhaling lavender oil provides the best remedy to stuffy sinuses.
- Topical- lavender essential oil is one of the few oils that can be used undiluted. Cleanse the affected area and drip one drop on it then allow it to air-dry.
- Bathing- lavender blends beautifully with many other essential oils and you can make your own bath and beauty products by taking advantage of its comforting fragrance.

Blending

Lavender essential oil blends well with bergamot, cedarwood, clary sage, clove, cypress, eucalyptus, geranium, german chamomile, grapefruit, lemon, lemongrass and many others. The list is very long!

Healing properties

It is ideal for treating depression, insect bites, insomnia, minor burns, minor cuts and scrapes, and sunburn.

2. **Clary Sage Essential Oil (*Salvia sclarea*)** Clary sage can do miracles to people who experience PMS or menopause symptoms. If you are looking for an essential oil that eases these symptoms, give clary sage a try. It has a component called sclareol, which acts similarly to

estrogen. It helps promote a sense of balanced calm in women. It also makes a perfect and uplifting blend to any mood-boosting regimen. Its scent is comforting and promotes a relaxed environment.

Precautions:

- Avoid using it when you are pregnant.
- Avoid topical use on children below 6 years.
- Consult your doctor before adding it to your regimen if on medication.

Application Methods:

- It can be inhaled, applied topically, or added to a bath.

Blending

Blends well with bergamot, cedarwood, clove, lemon, geranium, german chamomile, juniper berry, frankincense, ginger, grapefruit, lavender, tea tree, and more.

Healing properties

Clary sage essential oil is ideal for treating anxiety, body odor, depression, emotional upset, exhaustion, insomnia, menopause symptoms, painful periods, and PMS Stress.

3. **Lemon Essential Oil (*Citrus limonum*)** Lemon is a top ingredient in cleaning solutions. It shines in many

household cleaners. Its fragrance makes it versatile to blend well with many other essential oils. Lemon is like sunshine in a tiny bottle. Its ability to create a cheerful atmosphere can boost your mood when you feel dreary.

Precautions:

- Lemon essential oil can increase the likelihood of sunburn because of its phototoxic nature. Avoid direct exposure of the treated area to sunlight.

Application methods:

- Inhalation, topical, or added to a bath.

Blending
Lemon essential oil blends well with allspice, benzoin, caraway seed, cardamom, clove, eucalyptus, fennel seed, frankincense, geranium, ginger, grapefruit, lavender, lemongrass, orange, patchouli, peppermint, rosemary, tangerine, tea tree, and thyme.

Healing Properties
Lemon essential oils can treat allergies, asthma, athlete's foot, bronchitis, congestion, emotional upset, jock itch, nail fungus, respiratory infections, ringworm, and stress.

4. **Clove Essential Oil (*Syzygium aromaticum*)** Clove essential oil can boost your mood in a second, thanks to

its sweet scent. This sweet scent makes it ideal for homemade natural air-freshening blends. Clove is one of the best pain killers that even dentists used before the discovery of numbing agents.

Precautions:

- Never use it undiluted unless you are treating a toothache.
- Avoid using clove in pregnancy.
- Never use it if you have liver or kidney conditions.

Popular Uses:

- It is one of the best natural insect repellents.
- The best natural pain reliever for toothaches.

Application methods:

- inhalation, topical, and added to a bath.

Blending

Clove essential oil blends well with allspice, basil, benzoin, bergamot, cinnamon, clary sage, ginger grapefruit, helichrysum, hops, lavender, lemon, lime, orange, peppermint, and rosemary.

Healing properties

Clove essential oil can treat acne, athlete's foot, bad breath, body odor, bruises, cold and flu, cramping, headache, indigestion, insect bites and bee stings, jock itch, muscle pain, nail fungus, ringworm, sinusitis, and toothache.

5. **Eucalyptus Essential Oil (*Eucalyptus globulus*)** Eucalyptus essential oil is a fantastic addition to household natural air fresheners, thanks to its fresh and invigorating scent. When blended with essential oils like German chamomile, black pepper, clove bud, ginger, marjoram sweet, peppermint or rosemary, it creates a valuable pain-relieving synergy that makes it an important ingredient in many natural first-aid remedies. Its astringent properties reduce mucous membrane inflammation and is among the best essential oils for treating upper respiratory tract infections, and cold and flu symptoms.

Precautions:

- Avoid topical use on children under the age of 6 years.
- Don't use it if you are epileptic.
- Don't use it if you have high blood pressure.
- Overusing eucalyptus essential oils can contribute to headaches.

Uses:

- Can be used in remedies to help control fever.

- It aids in faster healing of compromised skin.

Application methods:

- Eucalyptus essential oil may be inhaled, applied topically, or added to baths.

Blending
It blends well with benzoin, cajuput, lavender, lemon, lemongrass, pine, rosemary, tea tree, and thyme.

Healing properties
Eucalyptus essential oil is ideal for treating asthma, blisters, burns, cold and flu, congestion, cuts and scrapes, headaches, insect bites and bee stings, sinusitis, and sunburn.

6. **Geranium (*Pelargonium odoratissimum*)** You likely will have come across geranium if you are a natural skincare product lover. The geranium essential oil has various properties that benefit itchy, dry, and aging skin. If you are a woman who wants to ease PMS and menopause symptoms, the geranium essential oil can be of great benefit; it offers gentle, hormone-balancing effects.

Precautions:

- Avoid using geranium essential oils if you are diabetic. It can lower blood sugar.

- Don't use it if you are pregnant.

Application methods:

- inhalation, topical, or added to a bath.

Uses:

- Can make hair shampoo and conditioner.
- Found in the various face, bath, and body products as it heals and nourishes the skin.
- Can also be used as a natural air freshener.

Blending

Geranium essential oil blends well with atlas cedar, bergamot, carrot seed, cedarwood, clary sage, cucumber seed, German chamomile, grapefruit, helichrysum, jasmine, juniper berry, lavender, lemon, lemongrass, lime, melissa, roman chamomile, and rosemary essential oils.

Healing properties

Geranium essential oil can be used for treating aging skin, anxiety, combination skin, dry skin, eczema, menopause symptoms, mild postnatal depression, mood swings, PMS symptoms, shingles, and stress.

7. **Grapefruit (*Citrus paradisi*)** Among all the citruses, grapefruit is the best mood-boosting essential oil; go for it

whenever you feel tired or in a funk. Its sweet, refreshing, pleasant fragrance makes it a perfect ingredient for creating a cheerful atmosphere in your home. A massage blend of grapefruit essential oil can help ease swollen feet and legs. Besides the amazing psychological effects, grapefruit is also a wonderful water retention remedy.

Precautions:

- Don't use grapefruit essential oil if you are taking statins or medicines that interact with grapefruit.
- Grapefruit essential oil can increase the likelihood of sunburn because of its phototoxic nature. Avoid direct exposure of the treated area to sunlight.

Application methods:

- inhalation, topical, and added to a bath.

Blending

Grapefruit essential oil blends well with bergamot, cardamom, cedarwood, cinnamon, clove, coriander, cypress, geranium, German chamomile, ginger, juniper berry, lavender, lemon, lime, mandarin, patchouli, peppermint, red mandarin, and Roman chamomile.

Healing properties

It can treat acne, anxiety, cellulite, depression, hangover, headache, fatigue, food cravings, menstrual cramps, mood swings, muscle cramps, muscle pain, oily skin, stress, and water retention.

8. **Frankincense Essential Oil (*Boswellia carterii, B. serrata, B. sacra*)** If you recall the nativity story of baby Jesus, frankincense was one of the three gifts that were brought to Jesus. Because of its spicy, warm, woody scent, it makes a classic ingredient for incense. It is very safe for babies. Besides its ability to heal rashes and relieve respiratory tract infections, frankincense essential oil offers a deep, calming influence that helps you to let go of stress.

Precautions:

- Don't use frankincense essential oil in pregnancy, or while breastfeeding.

Application methods:

- inhalation, added to a bath, and topical application.

Blending

Frankincense essential oil blends well with bergamot, black pepper, cinnamon, clove, cypress, geranium, grapefruit, helichrysum, lavender, lemon, mandarin, neroli, orange, palmarosa, patchouli, pine, geranium, vetiver, rose, and ylang-ylang.

Healing Properties

Frankincense essential oil is ideal for treating asthma, bronchitis, cold and flu symptoms, colic, gas, inflammation, laryngitis, minor cuts and scrapes, rashes, and scars.

9. **Peppermint Essential Oil (*Mentha piperita*)** You are likely to enjoy quick relief from tension headaches and migraines with peppermint essential oil. Thanks to its beautiful, fresh, intense minty aroma, it has many uses within beauty, cosmetics, aromatherapy, and soap-making. Peppermint essential oil is also an effective breath freshener.

Precautions:

- Avoid use on the face or chest of babies and children under the age of 6 years.
- Do not ingest peppermint essential oil. It can cause a serious adverse reaction.
- Do not overuse. It can lead to sensitization.
- Avoid using peppermint essential oil if breastfeeding.
- Avoid its use in pregnancy.
- It can irritate people with sensitive skin, do a patch test first before applying on the entire affected area.

Application methods:

- Inhalation, topical, and added to a bath.

Blending

Peppermint essential oil blends especially well with essential oils in the mint, wood, spice, citrus, and herbaceous families. Some of these oils include basil, benzoin, black pepper, catnip, cypress, eucalyptus, geranium, German chamomile, grapefruit, juniper, lavender, lemon, lemongrass, niaouli, orange, pine, rosemary, spearmint, tea tree, and thyme.

Healing properties

Peppermint essential oil is ideal for treating cold and flu symptoms, exhaustion, hangover, headaches, indigestion, insect bites and bee stings, itching, nausea, rashes, sunburn, and skin inflammation.

10. **Roman Chamomile (*Anthemis nobilis*)** Roman chamomile essential oil is one of the most expensive oils, but it is worth adding to your collection. Thanks to its soothing fragrance that combines a light floral and herbal aroma, it can soothe the body and mind alike, promoting peaceful sleep. Roman chamomile essential oil is also safe for infants.

Precautions:

- It may cause skin irritation to sensitive skin. Do a patch test first.
- Do not use while pregnant.

Application methods:

- inhalation, added to a bath, and topical application.

Blending
Roman chamomile essential oil blends well with bergamot, clary sage, eucalyptus, frankincense, geranium, grapefruit, helichrysum, hops, lavender, lemon, lemongrass, mandarin, patchouli, peppermint, rose, spearmint, tea tree, thyme, and ylang-ylang.

11. **Rosemary (*Rosmarinus officinalis*)** Rosemary essential oil has a wide range of uses that makes it exceptionally versatile. Its benefits range from easing cold and flu symptoms to relieving aches and pains. It is also an outstanding addition to hair care products, so, if you are concerned about hair loss, let it top your must-have essential oils list.

Precautions:

- Do not use it if you are pregnant.
- Don't use rosemary if you are epileptic.

Application Methods:

- inhalation, added to a bath, and topical use.

Blending

Rosemary essential oil blends perfectly with clary sage, clove, frankincense, geranium, grapefruit, lavender, lemon, lemongrass, pine, tea tree, thyme, basil, bay laurel, bergamot, and black pepper.

Healing properties

Rosemary essential oil can treat bronchitis, cold and flu symptoms, dandruff, fatigue, indigestion, nervousness, sinusitis, thinning hair, and varicose veins.

12. **Tea Tree (*Melaleuca alternifolia*)** Tea trees are sometimes referred to as melaleuca. It is one of the most widely respected and used essential oils. Because of its remarkable benefits in supporting optimal immune function and healthy skin and hair, tea tree essential oil is commonly used as an antibacterial, anti-inflammatory, antiviral, and for treating hypersensitivity. Tea tree essential oil has been praised in research and has proven to help wounds heal faster.

Precautions:

- Only use the inhalation method or apply it topically. Never ingest tea tree essential oil, no matter the purpose. It may cause dizziness, hives, or digestive issues.
- Do not use it undiluted.

Application methods:

- Inhalation, topical, and added to a bath.

Blending

Tea Tree essential oil blends well with lavender, peppermint, cinnamon, eucalyptus, juniper, niaouli, spikenard, clove, sandalwood, clay sage, and vetiver.

Healing Properties

Tea tree essential oil is ideal for treating acne, athlete's foot, body odor, cold and flu symptoms, dandruff, gingivitis, insect bites and bee stings, insect infestation, jock itch, minor burns, minor cuts and scrapes, nail fungus, oily skin and hair, ringworm, swimmer's ear, and yeast infections.

13. **Thyme Essential Oil (*Thymus vulgaris*)** Whenever you feel drained, reach out for thyme essential oil; its herbal scent provides a tremendous energy boost. Thyme essential oil offers a variety of benefits. Use it for an even skin tone or to relieve PMS and menopause symptoms. Thanks to its expectorant property, thyme helps relieve respiratory symptoms associated with cold and flu. Its ability to relieve joint and muscle pain makes it an outstanding addition to hot and cold compresses and balms and massage oils.

Precautions:

- Dilute it carefully before use.

- If you are allergic to peppermint or rosemary essential oil, thyme may also irritate you.
- Don't use it in pregnancy.
- Never use it topically on children below the age of 6 years.
- Avoid using it if you have hyperthyroidism.
- Avoid using it if you have high blood pressure, as it can elevate it.

Application methods:

- inhalation, added to a bath, and topical.

Blending
Thyme essential oil blends well with bergamot, black pepper, catnip, clary sage, geranium, grapefruit hyssop, juniper berry, lavender, lemon, lemongrass, lime, peppermint, pine, Roman chamomile, rosemary, spearmint, and tea tree.

Healing properties
It is ideal for treating aging skin, anxiety, cold, and flu symptoms, diarrhea, fatigue, hair loss, hangover, nervousness, PMS, stress, and upper respiratory infections.

14. **Patchouli (*Pogostemon cablin*)** Patchouli essential oil possesses an intriguingly sweet, earthy aroma with firm notes of wood and spice. Thanks to its remarkable fragrance, it can help serve as a natural fixative; it supports a peaceful mind, and acts as an insect repellent,

among many other uses. Aromatically, a little patchouli essential oil goes a long way. It is suited for both men and women.

Precautions:

- This is a safe essential oil

Application methods:

- inhalation, added to a bath, and topical.

Blending

It blends beautifully with many other essential oils and aromas especially those within the wood, citrus, floral, spicy, balsamic, and resinous families, such as bergamot, cinnamon, clary sage, clove, frankincense, geranium, German chamomile, ginger, grapefruit, lavender, lemon, lemongrass, lime, mandarin, myrrh, orange, rosemary, ylang-ylang, and yuzu.

Healing properties

Patchouli essential oil can treat athlete's foot, dandruff, depression, eczema, hemorrhoids, jock itch, nail fungus, ringworm, and yeast infection.

Chapter Four: Therapeutic Properties of Essential Oils

People from all walks of life have been using essential oils to improve their health since ancient times. In this chapter, we will explain how essential oils help to support healing the body, plus simple ways to harness the healing power of aromatherapy to address the most commonly treated ailments. Health and vitality depend on the harmonious and collective functioning of each organ in the body. That's why we have simplified everything by identifying and separating bodily systems and their association with various essential oils. And again, most essential oils treat multiple ailments. Therefore, we have divided the chapter to deal with the major systems of the body which include the digestive system, nervous system, circulatory system, respiratory system, reproductive system, musculoskeletal system, and urinary system.

The Circulatory System

The circulatory system comprises the heart, blood vessels, and lymph nodes. The heart and blood vessels transport blood throughout the body. The lymph nodes transport cellular fluids and nutrients.

High Blood Pressure: High blood pressure is a condition brought about by old age, stress, poor diet, and lack of exercise. When not attended to, it can cause serious problems like kidney failure, stroke, and even death. Regular aromatherapy massage with essential oils can help ease hypertension. Essential oils that are useful in normalizing blood pressure include clary sage, melissa, lavender, marjoram, ginger, Roman and German chamomile, valerian, vetiver, spikenard, orange, neroli, and ylang ylang.

For a massage to lower your blood pressure, simply dilute:

- 2 drops of marjoram
- 3 drops of lavender
- 3 drops of ylang ylang
- 20ml of carrier oil

Reynaud's syndrome: This is an interesting condition that results in poor blood circulation. Reynaud's syndrome is also brought about by stress. To improve general blood circulation, use infused oils from basil, rosemary, thyme, marjoram, and clove herbs. A sedating massage with the essential oils of melissa, neroli, lavender, and ylang-ylang that help relieve stress-related heart problems can also help to improve symptoms.

Try this as a massage blend:

- 4 drops of black pepper essential oil
- 1 drop of rosemary essential oil
- 3 drops of neroli (or rose)
- 20 ml of carrier oil

Varicose veins: This is a condition where the veins become distended because of too much blood (or lymph) pooling in the area (usually in the lower legs). Chamomile, myrtle, lemon, neroli, and cypress essential oils ease the inflammation and pain of varicose veins; frankincense essential oil helps constrict distended veins.

Try this blend:

- cypress essential oil, 6 drops
- myrtle essential oil, 3 drops
- German chamomile essential oil, 3 drops
- frankincense essential oil (optional), 2 drops
- 1 ounce St. John's wort–infused oil

The Digestive System

The effectiveness of how we process and assimilate nutrients and thoroughly eliminate waste largely influences our well-being. Digestion is closely linked to your sense of smell. Aromas play a role in the initial stage of digestion; they signal the brain, alerting it that food is on the way.

Constipation: To ease constipation, choose essential oils that are useful for easing muscle spasms and use the blend for a slow abdominal massage. Such essential oils include peppermint, geranium, black pepper, juniper, and fennel.

A useful massage blend can be:

- 3 drops of peppermint essential oil
- 2 drops of geranium essential oil
- 3 drops of juniper essential oil
- 20 ml of carrier oil

Diarrhea: With diarrhea, it is important to look into the underlying causes. If it is caused by food poisoning or infections, then essential oils with antibacterial properties and pain-relieving properties would help. Examples of such essential oils include tea tree, rosewood, and ginger.

Try the following blend in a warm compress:

- 1 drop of tea tree essential oil
- 1 drop of rosewood essential oil
- 1 drop of ginger essential oil
- 20 ml of carrier oil

Gum disease: A combination of myrrh and tea tree essential oils is the most appropriate treatment for gum disease. You can also try the following facial blend designed to relieve pain and inflammation if you don't like either of these essential oils:

- 1 drop of Roman chamomile essential oil
- 1 drop of nutmeg essential oil
- 2 drops of lavender essential oil
- 20 ml of carrier oil

Stomach ulcers: To ease pain and discomfort from stomach ulcers, you just need a gentle abdominal massage with essential oils. The choice of essential oils to be used depends on the cause of the ulcers. If they are stress-related, try essential oils meant for anxiety-like neroli, clary sage, fennel, peppermint, frankincense, rose, or geranium. If the ulcers are caused by bacteria (such as H. pylori), use antibacterial essential oils like tea tree, rosewood, sandalwood, cypress, or lavender.

The Nervous System

One of the most satisfying areas to treat with aromatherapy is the nervous system. The nervous system facilitates the intricate connection between mind and body. Mental and emotional responses carry a problem from one area of the body to another.

Anxiety: Neroli is the most effective essential oil for treating anxiety. Just inhale its fragrance and it will calm you in no time. Other useful essential oils for relieving anxiety include mandarin, tangerine, orange, Roman chamomile, lavender, rose, benzoin, sandalwood, cedarwood, cypress.

Depression: Try bergamot, Roman chamomile, lavender, melissa, clary sage, neroli, rose, or jasmine essential oils if you are stressed. Other essential oils that may help relieve depression include orange, mandarin, tangerine, lemon, grapefruit, geranium, cypress, myrrh.

For mild depression, try this blend:

- 4 drops of mandarin essential oil
- 2 drops of sandalwood essential oil
- 2 drops of rose essential oil
- in 20 ml of carrier oil

To relax and get some relief from depression, you can use this formula as a massage or bath oil:

- lavender essential oil, 2 drops
- neroli essential oil, 2 drops

- marjoram essential oil, 2 drops
- ylang-ylang essential oil, 2 drops
- chamomile essential oil, 2 drops
- clary sage essential oil, 2 drops
- 1 ounce carrier oil

Insomnia: For insomnia caused by mental agitation or overwork, essential oils like benzoin, clary sage, geranium, Roman chamomile, German chamomile, cedarwood, jasmine, lavender, mandarin, marjoram, neroli, orange, patchouli, petitgrain, rose, rosewood, sandalwood, spikenard, tangerine, valerian, vetiver, yarrow, ylang ylang can help you unwind. It is advisable to start with lavender if you have trouble sleeping.

Neuralgia: Using essential oils in a massage can help ease neuralgia or what we commonly call nerve pains. For neuralgia relief, try this formula:

- helichrysum essential oil, 5 drops
- chamomile essential oil, 3 crops
- marjoram essential oil, 2 drops
- lavender essential oil, 2 drops
- 1 ounce carrier oil

Musculoskeletal System

Bones and muscles give our bodies form and enable physical movements in the body. Many kinds of pain in our bones and muscles can be relieved with the help of essential oils.

Sprains and Strains

To relieve muscle strain, use this massage formula:

- 3 drops of black pepper essential oil
- 3 drops of lavender essential oil
- 2 drops of rosemary essential oil
- 20 ml of carrier oil

Osteoarthritis

For osteoarthritis massage, try the following formula:

- 3 drops of German chamomile essential oil
- 3 drops of lavender essential oil
- 2 drops of rosemary
- 20 ml of carrier oil

Rheumatoid arthritis

Try the following massage formula to ease rheumatoid arthritis:

- 3 drops of marjoram essential oil
- 3 drops of lemon essential oil
- 2 drops of Roman chamomile essential oil
- 20 ml of carrier oil.

General Pain Relief Formula

Combine the following ingredients to ease general pain in muscles and bones. Use this formula for a massage or add 1 tablespoon to a bath:

- helichrysum essential oil, 6 drops
- marjoram essential oil, 4 drops
- juniper essential oil, 2 drops
- birch or wintergreen essential oil, 4 drops
- chamomile essential oil, 3 drops
- lavender essential oil, 3 drops
- ginger essential oil, 3 drops
- 2 ounces of carrier oil

The Respiratory System

Irritation and infection of the ears, nose, and throat are the most experienced afflictions of the respiratory system. Most of these problems involve congestion which can be eased by inhaling essential oils like rosemary, hyssop, tea tree, eucalyptus, lavender, or peppermint.

Asthma: Asthmatic people suffer a constant battle with low-level congestion. With mild asthma, the use of essential oils may help ease the symptoms. Helpful essential oils to ease asthma include clary sage, eucalyptus, frankincense, geranium, lavender, lemon, peppermint, Roman chamomile, and thyme.

Try this clary sage formula:

- 2 tablespoons jojoba oil (you can use the carrier oil if jojoba isn't readily available)
- 30 drops clary sage essential oil

Apply 5 to 7 drops of the combination of the two essential oils on your chest and neck, inhaling deeply. Repeat as required.

For infants, try this homemade nasal inhalant formula:

- 2 drops eucalyptus essential oil
- 2 drops rosemary essential oil
- 1 drop peppermint essential oil
- 1 tablespoon rock salt

Bronchitis: Bronchitis may be caused by exposure to lung irritants, and bacterial or viral infection. Aromatherapy may help ease the discomfort and inflammation. Essential oils that may help ease bronchitis include clove, eucalyptus, frankincense, lavender, lemon, peppermint, rosemary, and thyme.

Try this frankincense-clove massage formula. The combination of these two essential oils offers antibacterial properties and soothes inflamed airways. If you don't want to apply it topically, you can still enjoy the same benefits by adding the blend to an essential oil inhaler or diffuser:

- 5 drops clove essential oil
- 20 drops frankincense essential oil
- ¼ cup jojoba oil (or any carrier oil on hand)

The Reproductive System

Problems involving the reproductive system are among the most common problems experienced by women. Using essential oils can help treat these problems.

Menstrual cramps

For menstrual cramp relief, try the following massage formula:

- lavender essential oil, 4 drops
- marjoram essential oil, 2 drops
- chamomile or clary sage essential oil, 2 drops
- geranium essential oil, 3 drops
- ginger essential oil, 1 drop
- 1 ounce carrier oil (infused oil of yarrow)

Yeast infections

To ease yeast infections, try the following:

- thyme essential oil, 1 drop
- German chamomile essential oil, 1 drop
- lavender essential oil, 1 drop
- tea tree essential oil, 2 drops
- palmarosa essential oil, 2 drops
- geranium essential oil, 1 drop
- 2 cups warm yarrow tea

Combine the above ingredients and gently douche two times a day.

Premenstrual Symptoms (PMS)

Aromatherapy can help ease moodiness and help with symptoms such as hot flashes, cramping, and nausea. Helpful essential oils that ease PMS include clary sage, frankincense, geranium, lavender, patchouli, Roman chamomile, rosemary, and thyme.

The Urinary System

The urinary system comprises the bladder and kidneys. It plays a big role in regulating the body's water content and salt balance as well as eliminating bodily waste. Essential oils like cedarwood, tea tree, bergamot, and fennel work as antiseptic diuretics to treat bladder infections.

Bladder Infections Relief Formula

Combine the following essential oils and massage the mixture over the bladder area twice a day:

- tea tree essential oil, 6 drops
- 2 drops thyme essential oil (or sandalwood can be a good substitute)
- 2 drops juniper essential oil
- 2 drops clove essential oil
- 2 drops oregano essential oil
- 1 ounce carrier oil (calendula is one of the best choices)

The Integumentary System

The integumentary system comprises the skin, and it is one of the most important and the largest systems in our body. Your skin is what someone sees first on your body. Therefore, infections of the skin cause discomfort of the highest levels and can lower an individual's self-esteem. The antibacterial, antifungal, antiviral, antiseptic, and germ-killing properties of essential oils help treat the skin, repair it, and encourage new cell growth and faster healing. The different essential oils that are helpful for skin conditions include tea tree, lavender, helichrysum, cistus, eucalyptus, geranium, sandalwood, lemon, pine, and rose.

Fungal Infections: The essential oils that treat fungal infections include tea tree, peppermint, lavender, eucalyptus, myrrh, palmarosa, and geranium. Simply dilute these essential oils with vinegar, soak a compress, and apply to the affected area.

You can also try the following fungal powder to keep the area dry. Combine the ingredients in a small bowl and liberally powder the affected area:

- bentonite clay, ¼ cup
- goldenseal root powder, 1 tablespoon
- tea tree essential oil , 12 drops
- clove essential oil , 12 drops
- geranium essential oil, 12 drops

Inflammation and Burns: Use anti-inflammatory essential oils such as chamomile, lavender, or marjoram for inflammation. Simply apply a cold compress of these oils to the affected areas. For burns and sunburns, quickly immerse the affected area in cold water containing few drops of these oils. Apply lavender or aloe vera essential oils to enhance new cell growth, reduce inflammation, and stop infections in the affected area.

Insect Bites and other Critter Attacks: A simple dab of lavender and tea tree essential oils provides relief from insect bites. To reduce swelling, itching, and inflammation, you can also use chamomile and lavender.

Chapter Five: Aromatherapy for Skin, Hair, and Nail Care

The condition of our face, hair, skin, and even nails reflect our inner health. Using essential oils to treat the face, skin, and hair is one of the most common and enjoyable uses of aromatherapy. It is also easy to develop aromatherapy treatments for these areas. This chapter looks at the different skin and hair types and suggests aromatherapy treatments for them.

Skin Care

The skin is the largest organ in your body. It handles many vital functions; it protects our internal organs, adjusts our body temperature, and it is also responsible for most sensations in our body. For you to treat the skin using essential oils effectively, you need to approach each type of skin differently.

Oily skin

Oily skin is usually shiny, sensitive, and is thicker and coarser than other skin types. Though your skin's natural oil provides protection from the elements and holds moisture in, excessively oily skin is prone to blackheads, whiteheads, clogged pores, and other blemishes. Helpful essential oils for this type of skin are those that are antiseptic and balance hormonal activity and the production of sebum. They include clary sage, clove, eucalyptus, geranium, grapefruit, lavender, lemon, lemongrass, patchouli, Roman chamomile, rosemary, tea tree, and thyme.

Try this formula:

- 3 drops of lemon essential oil
- 1 drop of juniper essential oil
- 4 drops of lavender essential oil
- 40 ml of cleanser

Dry skin

Dry skin feels tight with visible flaking in some areas. It is sensitive to cold, wrinkles easily, and occasionally feels rough to the touch. Dry skin can be irritatingly itchy. The good is news is that the use of balancing essential oils can reduce itching and flakiness while increasing softness and imparting a healthier appearance. Helpful essential oils for this include lavender, sandalwood, geranium, rose, neroli, Roman chamomile, clary sage, jasmine, patchouli, rosewood, sandalwood, ylang ylang, German chamomile, palmarosa.

Try this formula to make about 1 cup of Roman chamomile-frankincense facial moisturizer:

- 10 drops of frankincense essential oil
- 15 drops of Roman chamomile essential oil
- ½ cup of cocoa butter
- ½ cup of coconut oil
- 1½ teaspoons of apricot kernel oil
- 1½ teaspoons of rosehip oil (optional)
- 1 tablespoon of vegetable glycerin (optional)

Instructions:

- Combine the frankincense and Roman chamomile essential oils in a small bottle.

- Let the combination rest overnight.
- Combine the essential oils, cocoa butter, coconut oil, apricot kernel oil, rosehip oil, and glycerin in a clean, dry bowl or blender.
- Process or blend until the mixture becomes smooth.
- Transfer the blend to a clean, dry bowl, and refrigerate until firm.
- Whip the solidified cream with a handheld mixer until it gains a light, silky texture.
- Transfer the finished cream to a bottle with a tight-fitting lid.
- Apply about a pea-size amount of moisturizer on your face after washing it.
- Use it once or twice daily.

Dehydrated skin

This type of skin simply lacks water. It is characterized by reddening, dryness, flaking around the nostrils, broken blood vessels, or a chapped appearance. Apart from increasing water intake, the use of essential oils that heal the skin and balance out sebum production is key. Helpful essential oils include frankincense, benzoin, geranium, lavender, neroli, patchouli, rose, and sandalwood.

Try this formula to reduce the appearance of broken capillaries:

- 2 drops of cypress essential oil
- 1 drop of bergamot essential oil
- 1 drop of patchouli essential oil
- 20 ml of jojoba oil

Combination Skin

This type of skin can either be normal/dry or normal/oily. The appearance of the skin in the T-zone (forehead, nose, and chin) and the rest of the face is always different. You may have dry cheeks and an oily T-zone, for example. Helpful essential oils to treat this include clary sage, eucalyptus, frankincense, geranium, grapefruit, lavender, lemon, lemongrass, patchouli, Roman chamomile, and tea tree.

Try this formula:

- 8 drops of patchouli essential oil
- 4 drops of Roman chamomile essential oil
- ½ cup of sweet almond carrier oil
- ½ cup of sugar

The above combined make about 1 cup of sugar scrub. Apply it topically. It is safe for children 12 years and above.

Aging Skin

Aging skin is characterized by dryness, age spots, fine lines, and wrinkles. Aging skin needs special care. Essential oils that encourage collagen production, deliver antioxidants, and those that help you retain moisture can assist in restoring aging skin. Helpful essential oils include clary sage, frankincense, geranium, patchouli, Roman chamomile, and thyme.

Try the following formula:

- 24 drops frankincense essential oil
- ½ cup avocado oil

Instructions:

- Combine the two ingredients in a bottle or jar with a tight-fitting lid to form a moisturizing oil cleanse.
- Wet your face with warm water and apply about ½ teaspoon of the oil blend to your face.
- Massage in light, circular motions.
- Place a washcloth in warm water, wring it out well, and then place it over your face for about 15 seconds. Use it gently to remove excess oil.
- Pat your skin dry using a soft towel. Do this twice daily.

Scars

The appearance of scars and dark spots on your skin can be disturbing. Using essential oils can help you overcome this challenge. Helpful essential oils include clary sage, frankincense, geranium, lavender, patchouli, Roman chamomile, and tea tree.

Try this formula:

To make about ¼ a cup of frankincense–tea tree fading balm, combine:

- 8 drops frankincense essential oil
- 3 drops tea tree essential oil
- ¼ cup coconut oil, barely melted

Instructions:

- In a bottle or jar with a tight-fitting lid, combine the frankincense and tea tree essential oils.

- Let the mixture rest for at least 1 hour then use a chopstick or any other available thin utensil to stir the mixture in the coconut oil until blended completely.
- Apply a drop of balm to the scar using a cotton swab or your fingertips. Do this twice daily. Be patient, it may take several weeks to see the results.

Stretch Marks

Stretch marks are angry looking, indented, reddened streaks that appear on the skin when it stretches or shrinks quickly, especially during a period of rapid weight change. Even though it is difficult to completely prevent or remove stretch marks, the use of essential oils can often reduce their appearance and improve the skin's texture. The essential oils that can help reduce stretch marks include clary sage, frankincense, geranium, lavender, patchouli, Roman chamomile, and tea tree.

Try this formula to make about 1 cup of stretch mark balm:

- 10 drops of geranium essential oil
- 20 drops of lavender essential oil
- 10 drops of patchouli essential oil
- 10 drops of Roman chamomile essential oil
- ½ cup of cocoa butter
- ¼ cup of coconut oil
- ¼ cup of jojoba oil

Instructions:

- Combine the geranium, lavender, patchouli, and Roman chamomile essential oils in a small bottle.
- Let the combination rest overnight.

- Combine the cocoa butter and coconut oil in a double boiler over medium-low heat and stir until they are melted.
- Add the jojoba oil and the blended essential oils to the mixture.
- Transfer the liquefied blend to a small bowl and keep it in a refrigerator for 2 hours.
- Whip the solidified cream with a handheld mixer until it gains a light, silky texture.
- Transfer the balm to a bottle with a tight-fitting lid.
- Apply about ½ teaspoon of the cream to the affected areas. Use it at least twice a day.

Hair Care

There is nothing more radiant than beautiful, shiny, vibrant hair. Achieving shiny, healthy hair isn't that hard, but the hiked prices of conventional products that often contain unwanted chemicals are a great hindrance. With the help of nature's healing plants, keeping your hair beautiful is easy and fun. Next time you're looking for a good way to improve your hair's look and feel, try aromatherapy. Helpful essential oils for shiny, healthy hair include clary sage, clove, eucalyptus, geranium, grapefruit, lavender, lemon, lemongrass, patchouli, peppermint, Roman chamomile, rosemary, tea tree, thyme.

Normal hair

If your hair is "normal", then what you're currently using on it is likely just fine. However, be careful to check the label for the pH, harmful, or artificial ingredients. Helpful essential oils for normal hair are lavender and rosemary.

Oily hair

Excess sebum production, which is a condition that causes oily skin, also causes oily hair. Excess oil in the hair makes it look heavy and lifeless. People with this type of hair would want to wash it repeatedly with harsh shampoos that strip away all the oil. Though the short-term results might be good, your scalp goes into overdrive, prompting the sebaceous glands to manufacture more oil. The essential oils that can help keep your hair looking its best are clary sage, clove, eucalyptus, geranium, grapefruit, lavender, lemon, lemongrass, patchouli, Roman chamomile, rosemary, tea tree, thyme.

Dry hair

If you have a dry type of skin, then your air is likely also dry. The keratin protein your hair contains turns brittle when it is dry. Such hair becomes vulnerable to split ends and can produce flakes and appear unmanageable. Conditioning herbs for dry hair include calendula, chamomile, lavender, rosemary, and sandalwood.

Aromatic Hair Treatments

Use these natural hair treatments to gain clean and healthy hair.

Scalp Treatment

To treat dandruff and falling hair, or to stimulate hair growth, use this recipe:

- 25 drops of essential oil (cedarwood, geranium, juniper, sage, spearmint, tea tree, rosemary, or any essential oil suitable for healthy hair).

- 2 ounces of carrier oil (witch hazel, aloe juice, jojoba oil, or neem oil).
- Combine the ingredients and apply to the scalp. Massage it in, and then leave the treatment on for 1 to 2 hours before you shampoo it out.

Lice Treatment

To thoroughly eliminate lice and hatching eggs, use the following formula. Always do a patch test first as this is a strong solution:

- 20 drops of eucalyptus essential oil
- 10 drops of rosemary essential oil
- 10 drops of juniper essential oil
- 20 drops of lavender essential oil
- 10 drops of geranium essential oil
- 5 drops of ylang-ylang essential oil
- 4 ounces carrier oil (soy or coconut is best)

Combine the ingredients and apply to dry hair. Cover with a shower cap. Wrap the head in a towel to prevent vapors from irritating the eyes. Leave the treatment on for 1 to 2 hours and then shampoo it out. For effective results, repeat the treatment every 3 days for a total of 3 treatments.

Hair-Growth Formula

For an effective hair growth formula, combine the following ingredients and put them in a dark-colored bottle with a tight lid. Shake well and massage into the scalp for 10 minutes. Use it every night:

- 50 drops (½ teaspoon) of rosemary essential oil
- ½ cup aloe vera gel
- 1 tablespoon of apple cider vinegar
- 1 tablespoon of jojoba oil

Nail Care

Some people don't give their nails the attention and care they deserve. They abuse, chew, and neglect them. For you to have healthy nails, you need to give them good care. Gentle shaping, moisturizing, and buffing encourage just that. Combining these things with herbal and essential oil treatments will provide the best results! Helpful herbal and essential oils for nail care include tea tree, geranium, cinnamon, lavender, sandalwood, bay laurel, comfrey root, oat straw, and horsetail.

Antifungal Nail Oil

If you don't mind the smell of tea tree oil, you can use it by itself for this oil. Just be careful not to rub it in your eyes. Apply this around and under the nail 3 times daily:

- 5 drops of tea tree or geranium essential oil
- 1 drop of cinnamon bark essential oil
- in ½ ounce neem oil (or calendula-infused oil)

Aromatic Nail-Conditioning Soak

If you have dry or torn cuticles, this soak is best for you.

Combine the following:

- 2 drops of lavender essential oil
- 2 drops of bay laurel essential oil
- 2 drops of sandalwood essential oil
- in ½ ounce jojoba or neem oil

Put the mixture in a bowl and soak your nails in for 10 minutes. Buff to stimulate circulation and bring out a healthy shine.

Chapter Six: Aromatherapy Massage

There is nothing more calming and rejuvenating than a good massage at the end of a stressful, hard workday. As Hippocrates said, "The way to health is to have an aromatic bath and a scented massage every day."

As discussed in the previous chapters, some essential oils may be inhaled, and others may be absorbed in the body through the skin (massage). An aromatherapy massage is one of the simplest and most effective ways of using essential oils. Whilst the magic and the creativity of aromatherapy might be in the blending, the care and the therapeutic value of the massage application cannot be underestimated. This chapter discusses the benefits of aromatherapy massage, guidelines for performing it, and the different standard massage strokes.

Benefits of Aromatherapy Massage
- It plays a big role in relaxing both the mind and body.
- It helps in the relief of pain.
- Aromatherapy massage improves sleep.
- Aromatherapy massage enhances rejuvenation.
- It relieves headaches caused by tension.
- Aromatherapy massage stimulates the lymphatic system, thus removing toxins from the body.
- Aromatherapy massage helps reduce stress-related symptoms.
- It also nourishes the skin, giving it a healthy look when the oil is massaged in.
- Aromatherapy massage also helps soften the fat deposits.

Safety Tips for Aromatherapy Massage

- Be careful when performing the massage near open flames, as the oils used in aromatherapy are flammable.
- Ensure that the oils are lightly scented. A smell that is too strong quickly overwhelms both the person giving the massage and the one receiving it.
- For standard massage oil, we suggest a dilution of 2 percent of essential oil in a carrier oil.
- Lower dilutions may be more appropriate when performing a lymph-drainage massage or another type of bodywork requiring lots of oil.
- A 3 percent dilution is sufficient for a liniment which must be more concentrated to work properly.
- Never use painful pressure during an aromatherapy massage.
- Avoid massaging bones directly as it may cause injuries.
- Individuals who are pregnant or who have stomach problems should not have their abdominal areas massaged.
- Individuals undergoing any chemotherapy are not fit for aromatherapy massage.
- For individuals who are epileptic, or prone to any other type of seizure, a massage shouldn't be performed without a doctor's approval.
- Individuals who have or may have blood clots are not suitable candidates for an aromatherapy massage.
- Individuals who are under care for high blood pressure or have a heart condition of any kind are not fit for an aromatherapy massage.
- Individuals who are diabetic should consult their doctors before proceeding with an aromatherapy massage.
- If an individual has any form of rash or dermatitis, do not proceed with an aromatherapy massage.

- Forgo any massage in individuals with full-body acne. The risks of spreading the infection through the entire system are high.
- For individuals with fungus under their fingernails or toenails, it is advisable that they seek medical assistance and get it cleared up before performing a massage.

Standard Massage Movements

Aromatherapy massage can be performed using any method of hand movement. It requires long, slow strokes alternating with fast friction rubs while always maintaining contact with the body. The friction rubs warm the oils and helps spread them evenly over the skin. Greater pressure should apply to the heavier muscle areas like the buttocks, shoulders, and back. The abdomen, pelvic region, and bony areas are among the delicate areas, and therefore, these areas should be stroked lightly. Below is a simple guide to the different massages and the basic massage movements required for aromatherapy massage to achieve the best results.

Effleurage (Stroking Movements)

This is the most popular massage movement. It involves a series of gentle strokes, enabling the massage oil to penetrate the body, helping to bring about a state of calm and relaxation. When doing Effleurage movements, you use the flat portion of the palms and fingers to exert even pressure on all the parts of your hand. Use your entire hands to perform short or long full strokes. The pressure used may be firm or gentle, depending on how you feel.

Effleurage is a very flexible type of massage, as it can be used both in extensive areas like the back or legs and in small areas like the cheeks of the face.

This type of massage has tremendous stress-reducing effects on the body, including:

- Minimized overall tension
- Calmed and soothed nerve endings
- Relaxation of muscle groups
- Rebalanced blood flow and increased circulation

Petrissage (Kneading Movements)

Try to imagine the motion your hands make when kneading a mound of dough; it is the same movement for petrissage massage. The movement should not look like you are attacking the body, causing pain and discomfort. Rather, it should be performed slowly and carefully. The most receptive areas to this kind of massage include the fat-collecting parts, like the thighs, stomach, and back. It can also be applied to muscular areas.

Petrissage, when done properly, can:

- Relax overworked muscles
- Release trapped toxins
- Increase circulation
- Aid the flow of lymphatic fluids

If you are a beginner, put slight pressure on your thumb while performing kneading movements. Do this until you improve your techniques to the point where all five fingers are exerting even amounts of pressure in unison.

1. **Friction or "Frottage" (Circular Movements):** This type of movement is beneficial to cold areas or those with poor circulation specifically. It involves rubbing the skin with the flat of the hand, in fast circular motions.

2. **Tapotement Movements:** This type of massage technique involves soft, rapid, striking movements from the wrists of the masseur. This movement can be used on the face, especially in the areas around the eyes and mouth. It follows the action your fingers would take over piano keys, which is why some people call this movement the "piano" motion.

3. **Pummeling Movements:** To perform this type of movement, make one or both of your hands into fists. Bounce the fits up and down the area in a fast, drumming movement while keeping your fingers held in. You can also carry out pummeling with flat hands, and fingertips down or with palms turned upwards. The sides of the hands can also perform pummeling movements.

4. **Fanning:** Fanning movements work best on the back, chest, legs, and arms. They help stretch and manipulate tension away from muscles. To perform this fanning movement, create a three-stroke fan shape from a single point and do an outward stroking motion as if you are combing the flesh with the backs of the fingers, using your nails.

5. **Chopping:** Chopping is another motion that works perfectly on the back of the shoulder blades and the back of the legs. To perform this movement, rotate the outer edge of your both hands up and down over the area. This movement is not meant for the timid because it is very vigorous. To do it properly, put in a lot of energy.

Massaging Specific Areas

Kindly note that the following ideas are not the only way to perform a full-body massage. However, if you are a beginner, they are a good place to start.

Neck massage

To massage the neck, use effleurage movements. To perform an effective neck massage, start at the base of the neck and move gently in a circular motion towards the base of the occipital bone. Be careful not to put pressure on the vertebrae to avoid injuries.

Feet Massage

When massaging the feet, begin from the toes moving in an upward direction to the ankle. Keep your thumbs on the sole of the feet with the fingers on top if somebody else is doing it for you. If you are doing it by yourself, have your thumbs on top with your fingers underneath.

The Legs

The legs can be massaged using effleurage, petrissage, and chopping movements. Always do the massage in an upward motion, starting from the ankles to the thighs using effleurage strokes. This calms tired legs. Use petrissage on the fatty or muscular areas like the thighs.

The Arms

For the arm massage, use petrissage movements. Using upward strokes, knead on the muscles on the forearm to the biceps of the upper arm. Use either one or both hands to do it.

The Shoulders

The chosen massage movements for the shoulders are effleurage and petrissage. Most people hold a lot of stress in their shoulders. Use petrissage movements to knead the muscles from the outer edges towards the center. Here, you are supposed to use both hands and the force of your actions should come from your thumbs and palms.

The Back

Combining chopping, effleurage, or petrissage movements for the back massage is very helpful in keeping your fingers and hands from tiring too quickly. In all the movements, it is always important to apply firm pressure.

Begin from the lower back, moving upwards towards the top of the shoulders and then back down the sides of the back if you decide to start with effleurage. Stop at the shoulder blade and perform several chopping movements. Follow this movement by kneading the sides of the back.

The Abdomen

Using effleurage strokes in circular movements in a clockwise direction is the most recommended way to massage your abdomen. To massage the lower abdomen and hips, start from the lower back and slide over the hips, then to the abdomen using effleurage strokes. Use your whole flat hand against your skin while performing these strokes.

Chapter Seven: Charts

The following charts present a summary of the information discussed in this book in an easy-to-use format. The most creative and interesting part of aromatherapy is designing your own homemade blends. This is because you can add your own intention to them.

These charts will serve as a quick reference guide to help you choose the best essential oils for your blends.

Essential Oils, Category, & Best Blends

Essential Oil	Category	Blends Well With
Lavender	Middle note	Bergamot, Cedarwood, Clary sage, Clove, Cypress, Eucalyptus, Geranium, German chamomile, Grapefruit, Lemon, and Lemongrass.
Clary Sage	Top note	Bergamot, Cedarwood, Clove, Lemon, Geranium, German chamomile, Juniper berry, Frankincense, Ginger, Grapefruit, Lavender, and Tea tree.
Lemon	Top note	Allspice, Benzoin, Caraway seed, Cardamom, Clove, Eucalyptus,

		Fennel seed, Frankincense, Geranium, Ginger, Grapefruit, Lavender, Lemongrass, Orange, Patchouli, Peppermint, Rosemary, Tangerine, Tea tree, and Thyme.
Clove	Top note	Allspice, Basil, Benzoin, Bergamot, Cinnamon, Clary sage, Ginger, Grapefruit, Helichrysum, Hops, Lavender, Lemon, Lime, Orange, Peppermint, and Rosemary.
Eucalyptus	Top note	Benzoin, Cajuput, Lavender, Lemon, Lemongrass, Pine, Rosemary, Tea tree, and Thyme.
Geranium	Middle note	Atlas cedar, Bergamot, Carrot seed, Cedar wood, Clary sage, Cucumber seed, German chamomile, Grapefruit, Helichrysum, Jasmine, Juniper berry, Lavender, Lemon, Lemongrass, Lime, Melissa, Roman chamomile, and Rosemary.
Grapefruit	Middle note	Bergamot, Cardamom, Cedar wood, Cinnamon, Clove, Coriander, Cypress, Geranium, German chamomile, Ginger,

		Juniper berry, Lavender, Lemon, Lime, Mandarin, Patchouli, Peppermint, Red mandarin, and Roman chamomile.
Frankincense	Base note	Bergamot, Black pepper, Cinnamon, Clove, Cypress, Geranium, Grapefruit, Helichrysum, Lavender, Lemon, Mandarin, Neroli, Orange, Palmarosa, Patchouli, Pine, Rose, Geranium, Vetiver, and Ylang-Ylang.
Peppermint	Top note	Basil, Benzoin, Black pepper, Catnip, Cypress, Eucalyptus, Geranium, German chamomile, Grapefruit, Juniper, Lavender, Lemon, Lemongrass, Niaouli, Orange, Pine, Rosemary, Spearmint, Tea tree, and Thyme.
Roman Chamomile	Middle note	Bergamot, Clary sage, Eucalyptus, Frankincense, Geranium, Grapefruit, Helichrysum, Hops, Lavender, Lemon, Lemongrass, Mandarin, Patchouli, Peppermint, Rose, Spearmint, Tea tree, Thyme, and Ylang-Ylang.
Rosemary	Middle note	Clary sage, Clove, Frankincense,

		Geranium, Grapefruit, Lavender, Lemon, Lemongrass, Pine, Tea tree, Thyme, Basil, Bay laurel, Bergamot, and Black pepper.
Tea Tree	Top note	Lavender, Peppermint, Cinnamon, Eucalyptus, Juniper, Niaouli, Spikenard, Clove, Sandalwood, Clay sage, and Vetiver.
Thyme	Top note	Bergamot, Black pepper, Catnip, Clary sage, Geranium, Grapefruit, Hyssop, Juniper berry, Lavender, Lemon, Lemongrass, Lime, Peppermint, Pine, Roman chamomile, Rosemary, Spearmint, and Tea tree.
Patchouli	Base note	Bergamot, Cinnamon, Clary sage, Clove, Frankincense, Geranium, German chamomile, Ginger, Grapefruit, Lavender, Lemon, Lemongrass, Lime, Mandarin, Myrrh, Orange, Rosemary, Ylang-Ylang, and Yuzu.
Lemongrass	Top note	Clary sage, Clove, Coriander, Cypress, Eucalyptus, Geranium, Ginger, Grapefruit, Lavender, Lemon, Patchouli, Peppermint, Rosemary, Tea Tree, and Thyme.
Basil	Top note	Bergamot, Fennel, Geranium, Grapefruit, Juniper, and Lavender.

Bergamot	Top note	Cypress, Jasmine, Lavender, Neroli, Patchouli, and Ylang-Ylang.
Parsley	Base note	Cypress, Geranium, Grapefruit, and Sage.
Ylang-ylang	Base note	Bergamot, Clary sage, Frankincense, Jasmine, Lavender, Lemon, and Neroli.

Essential Oils & Therapeutic Properties

Essential Oil	Therapeutic Properties
Basil	Treats: muscle pain, colds, depression, fatigue.
Bergamot	Acts as: antidepressant, antiparasitic, anti-inflammatory.
Benzoin	Treats: bacterial infections, inflammation, lung/ sinus congestion.
Black pepper	Treats: circulation/blood pressure problems, indigestion, lung/sinus congestion, pain/muscle cramps, viral infections, bacterial infections, fungal infections.
Cedar wood	Treats: Bacterial infections, lung/sinus congestion.
Cinnamon	Treats: headaches, bacterial infections, fungal infections, indigestion, pain/muscle cramps, viral infections.
Chamomile	Treats: diaper rash, earache, eczema, heartburn, indigestion, infant teething, insomnia, nausea, stress.
Clary Sage	Treats: anxiety, body odor, depression, emotional upset, exhaustion, insomnia, menopause symptoms, painful periods, PMS discomfort, stress, muscular pain.
Clove	Treats: acne, athlete's foot, bad breath, body

	odor, bruises, cold and flu, cramping, headache, indigestion, insect bites and bee stings, jock itch, muscle pain, nail fungus, ringworm, sinusitis, toothache.
Cypress	Acts as: an astringent, circulation stimulant, antiseptic.
Eucalyptus	Acts as: decongestant, antiviral, antibacterial, stimulant. Treats: asthma, blisters, burns, cold and flu, congestion, cuts and scrapes, headaches, insect bites and bee stings, sinusitis, sunburn.
Fennel	Treats: hormonal imbalances, indigestion, bacterial infections, inflammation, lung/sinus congestion.
Frankincense	Treats: asthma, bronchitis, cold and flu symptoms, colic, gas, inflammation, laryngitis, minor cuts and scrapes, rashes, scars.
Geranium	Treats: aging skin, anxiety, combination skin, dry skin, eczema, menopause symptoms, mild postnatal depression, mood swings, PMS symptoms, shingles, stress.
Ginger	Treats: blood pressure/circulation, indigestion, headache, lung/sinus congestion, menstrual issues, pain/muscle cramps, bacterial infections.

Grapefruit	Treats: acne, anxiety, cellulite, depression, hangover, headache, fatigue, food cravings, menstrual cramps, mood swings, muscle cramps, muscle pain, oily skin, stress, water retention.
Helichrysum	Acts as: antibacterial, antifungal, anti-inflammatory, and eases pain/muscle cramps.
Hyssop	Acts as: antibacterial, antiviral, and eases lung/sinus congestion.
Jasmine	Acts as: aphrodisiac. Treats: muscular pain.
Juniper berry	Treats: skin issues, PMS, stress, muscular pain, lung/sinus congestion.
Lavender	Acts as: antiviral, antibacterial, antidepressant, anti-inflammatory, antispasmodic. Treats: depression, insect bites, insomnia, minor burns, minor cuts and scrapes, sunburns.
Lemon	Treats: allergies, asthma, athlete's foot, bronchitis, congestion, emotional upset, jock itch, nail fungus, respiratory infections, ringworm, stress.

Lemon grass	Treats: athlete's foot, headache, jet lag, jock itch, nail fungus, ringworm, stress, yeast infection.
Marjoram	Acts as: antispasmodic, anti-inflammatory, antiseptic.
Melissa	Treats: circulation/blood pressure problems, headaches, indigestion, inflammation, bacterial infections, fungal infections, viral infections.
Myrrh	Treats: skin problems, inflammation, indigestion, bacterial infections, fungal infections, viral infections.
Neroli	Treats: circulation/blood pressure problems, inflammation, hormonal imbalances, viral and fungal infections.
Orange	Treats: circulation/blood pressure problems, indigestion, bacterial and viral infections.
Palmarosa	Treats: indigestion, depression, anxiety, fever, stress, trauma, nervous exhaustion.
Patchouli	Treats: athlete's foot, dandruff, depression, eczema, hemorrhoids, jock itch, nail fungus, ringworm, yeast infection.
Peppermint	Treats: cold and flu symptoms, exhaustion, hangover, headaches, indigestion, insect bites

	and bee stings, itching, nausea, rashes, sunburn, skin inflammation.
Rose	Acts as: aphrodisiac. Treats: indigestion, menstrual problems, bacterial, viral and fungal infections.
Rosemary	Treats: bronchitis, cold and flu symptoms, dandruff, fatigue, indigestion, nervousness, sinusitis, thinning hair, varicose veins.
Rosewood	Treats: eczema, wrinkles, stretchmarks, acne, bacterial, fungal and viral infections.
Sage	Treats: hormonal imbalances, menstrual problems, bacterial and viral infections.
Sandalwood	Acts as: aphrodisiac, anti-stress, anti-depressant. Treats: PMS.
Spearmint	Treats: indigestion, nausea, vomiting,

	common cold, headaches, muscle pain.
Tea tree	Treats: acne, athlete's foot, body odor, cold and flu, dandruff, gingivitis, insect bites and bee stings, insect infestation, jock itch, minor burns, minor cuts and scrapes, nail fungus, oily skin and hair, ringworm, swimmer's ear, yeast infections.
Thyme	Treats: aging skin, anxiety, cold and flu symptoms, diarrhea, fatigue, hair loss, hangover, nervousness, PMS, stress, upper respiratory infections.
Ylang ylang	Acts as: sleep aid, anti-stress, aphrodisiac, anti-bacterial, anti-viral Treats: headaches, circulation/blood pressure problems, PMS.

Conclusion

Thank you for reading this book all about aromatherapy!

By now, you should have a good understanding of what aromatherapy is, its long and storied history, and what different things it can be used to treat.

All that is left now is for you to take the next step, purchase some essential oils and carrier oils, and begin testing out aromatherapy for yourself! Whether you want to treat a specific physical ailment, or if you simply want to relax at the end of a long day, aromatherapy can do it all!

Thanks again for taking the time to read this book. I wish you the best of luck in your aromatherapy endeavors!

www.ingramcontent.com/pod-product-compliance
Lightning Source LLC
Chambersburg PA
CBHW060255030426
42335CB00014B/1714